I0093103

Sacred Space

52-Week Mental Health Journal for Women

Sacred Space

52-Week Mental Health Journal for Women

Create Daily Calm, Build Self-Worth, and Embrace Wellness with a Gentle Guided Journal for Reflection, Healing and Inner Strength

Aria Capri Publishing
Devon Abbruzzese
Mauricio Vasquez

The original purchaser of this book has permission to reproduce the pages of this book for personal use only. No other parts of this publication may be reproduced in whole or in part, shared with others, stored in a retrieval system, digitized, or transmitted in any form without written permission from the publisher.

Copyright 2025, Aria Capri Publishing (Aria Capri International Inc). All rights reserved.

Authors:
Aria Capri Publishing
Devon Abbruzzese
Mauricio Vasquez

First Printing: July 2025

ISBN - 978-1-998729-63-0 (Hardcover Book)
ISBN - 978-1-998729-62-3 (Paperback)

FREE BONUS

Enjoy a Free Digital Copy of This Transformational Journal—My Gift to You

Thank you for showing up for yourself and taking this powerful step toward daily self-care, reflection, and personal growth.

As a heartfelt gift, I'm offering you a FREE digital copy of THIS IS MY WAY: 365 Positive Thoughts and Self-Care Journal.

It's packed with inspiring messages and thought-provoking questions to help you build confidence, reduce anxiety, and reconnect with what matters most —all year long.

Claim your free e-copy by scanning this QR code:

Prefer a Physical Copy?

Many readers love having a physical copy to hold, highlight, or gift to someone special. If that sounds like you, you can grab your printed copy here:

Buy the hardcover version on Amazon by scanning this QR code:

Thank you for allowing me to be a small part of your self-care journey.

Here's to a year of reflection, growth, and positive change.

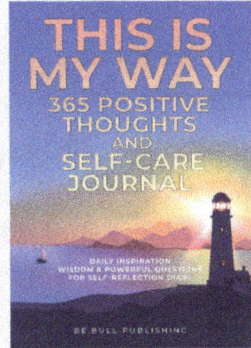

A Small Favor That Makes a Big Impact

If this journal has helped you pause, reflect, reconnect, or grow in even the smallest way—I'd be deeply grateful if you'd consider leaving a review.

As an independent author, I rely on the honest words of readers like you to help others discover this book. Your feedback not only supports the continued life of this work—it also reminds me why these quiet moments of reflection matter, one person and one page at a time.

You can share your thoughts by scanning the QR code. It only takes a minute, but your words have the power to help someone else begin their own journaling journey.

Thank you, truly, for being part of this. Your time, voice, and support mean more than you know.

Devon

Want More Journals and Resources?

Whether you're enjoying this journal and want to explore more titles, or you're looking for a digital version you can use on your device, you've got options!

📚 Print On Demand Store – Physical Copies

Use this QR code to visit our Amazon store and order printed editions of our books.

📥 Gumroad Store – PDF Versions at a Lower Price

Scan this QR code to access our Gumroad store, where you can purchase downloadable PDF versions of our books at a lower price— perfect for printing at home or using digitally.

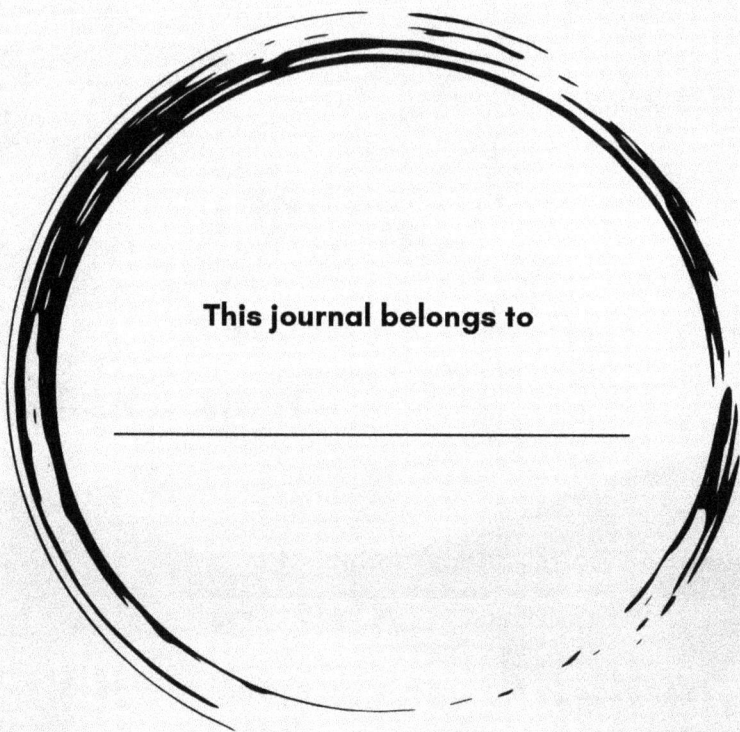

This journal belongs to

_____

Disclaimer

This journal is intended for personal reflection and general mental wellness support. It is not a substitute for professional advice, diagnosis, or treatment.

If you are experiencing emotional distress, a mental health crisis, or any situation that feels overwhelming, please seek guidance from a licensed physician, counselor, psychologist, or qualified mental health professional.

The author and publisher do not assume responsibility for any actions taken or not taken based on the content of this book. Use of this journal is entirely at the reader's discretion.

Your well-being matters—please reach out for professional help when needed.

Introduction

You're here. That matters. You've just made space for yourself—and that's a powerful choice.

This journal was created for women who give so much to others and sometimes forget to give back to themselves. If you've been running on empty, stuck in survival mode, or simply longing for a few quiet minutes to breathe, this is your invitation to pause... and listen inward.

Over the next 52 weeks, you'll gently return to yourself through short, compassionate prompts that support emotional renewal, clarity, and steadiness. Each week rotates through one of four healing foundations:

Calm and Resiliency, Connection and Engagement, Healthy Living, and Goals and Purpose.

You don't need to write the "right" answers. You don't need to dive deep every day. This is a flexible, no-pressure space.

Some days, you may write pages. Other days, a single sentence. Both are enough. What matters is showing up for yourself, even if it's just for five minutes.

This journal won't add to your to-do list—it will soften it. It won't demand energy—it will help you restore it. Think of it as a warm exhale at the end of the day. A permission slip to feel, reflect, and remember that you are worth tending to.

🌿 Calm and Resiliency

So many women carry stress silently—holding others up while forgetting to care for their own nervous systems.

This section helps you create small, steady moments of calm—without needing to escape your life. Through gentle reflection, you'll explore what soothes you, what strengthens your sense of safety, and what helps you return to center when life feels overwhelming.

Resilience doesn't mean being strong all the time. It means learning how to recover gently. It means noticing when you need a pause, and giving yourself permission to take it. These prompts are here to support that soft strength—the kind that rebuilds you slowly, kindly, and on your terms.

🌷 Connection and Engagement

You were never meant to carry it all alone.

Connection is a life force. But when caregiving, exhaustion, or emotional overload take center stage, relationships can fray—especially the one you have with yourself.

This section invites you to reflect on who you trust, who lights you up, and what it means to be fully seen. It also helps you reconnect with small joys—those moments of playfulness, beauty, or shared laughter that make life feel vibrant.

You'll gently explore how to engage with the world in ways that feel nourishing, not draining. And if you've been feeling disconnected or isolated, these prompts can help you find your way back—one word, one gesture, one moment at a time.

🌼 Healthy Living

True health is more than green smoothies or step counts. It's about listening to your body. Honoring its rhythms. And noticing how physical care fuels emotional steadiness.

This section explores everyday well-being—without judgment or rigid routines. You'll reflect on the small choices that help you feel more energized, rested, or emotionally balanced. That might mean choosing rest over hustle, or feeding your spirit as much as your body.

You'll also explore the connection between mind and body—how stress shows up physically, how joy brings ease, and how routines of care (like sleep, movement, or stillness) can restore your sense of vitality. The goal isn't perfection. It's reconnection—with the woman you're becoming when you take care of yourself like someone you love.

🌸 Goals and Purpose

Sometimes purpose feels crystal clear. Other times, it feels buried under exhaustion, doubt, or busyness.

This section is about gently rediscovering what matters to you. Not what's expected of you—but what's calling you forward. You'll reflect on what brings you meaning, what gives your days direction, and how to set goals that align with your values—not just your responsibilities. Whether you're starting something new, adjusting to change, or reclaiming your own dreams, these prompts help you reconnect with your inner compass.

You don't need to "have it all together." You just need a little space to listen to yourself and start again—with care.

✿ How to Use This Journal

Start any day you like. Keep this journal somewhere that feels inviting—your nightstand, your kitchen corner, your favorite chair.

There's no wrong way to journal. Write when you can. Skip a day if you need. Come back when you're ready. Your presence —not perfection—is what matters here.

Each daily prompt is short, supportive, and rooted in therapeutic insight. You'll find an easeful rhythm with time. And you may be surprised at how quickly you begin to feel clearer, steadier, and more emotionally connected.

This is your space to be honest, gentle, messy, quiet, bold— whatever you need today. There are no rules here, only invitations.

WEEK 1

Calm and Resiliency

1. Imagine you had three wishes granted overnight. What feelings come up when you picture that?

_____

_____

_____

_____

_____

2. When you think about those wishes, are there any that feel possible to begin exploring in real life?

_____

_____

_____

_____

_____

3. What brings you joy in your daily life—and how often do you make time for it?

....

....

....

....

....

4. What are you naturally good at? How might those strengths support your growth this year?

....

....

....

....

....

5. Is there a phrase or sentence you can say to yourself when things feel overwhelming?

....

....

....

....

....

6. What habits or sources of support help you get through difficult times with more care and kindness toward yourself?

....

....

....

....

....

7. How do you wind down and recharge at the week's end?

....

....

....

....

....

Connection and Engagement

1. What helps you feel connected to people you care about during the week?

....

....

....

....

....

2. If a kind friend wrote you a letter today, what would they say? How can you hold that message close?

....

....

....

....

....

3. Who do you feel better after talking to, and what makes those conversations feel meaningful?

....

....

....

....

....

4. Is there someone you miss? What would it take to reconnect in a way that feels safe and natural?

....

....

....

....

....

5. Think back to the last time you laughed with a friend. What made it special or memorable?

....

....

....

....

....

6. Who are two friends you appreciate? What would you say if you wrote them a simple note of gratitude?

....

....

....

....

....

7. What's something small you could do each day this week to share time or laughter with others?

....

....

....

....

....

Healthy Living

1. What shifts—big or small—would help your lifestyle feel more supportive and balanced?

....

....

....

....

....

2. What's one small step you could take to begin making those changes happen?

....

....

....

....

....

3. What does taking good care of your body look like for you right now? What's helping?

....

....

....

....

....

4. What's been weighing on you lately—and what have you done to lighten the load?

....

....

....

....

....

5. Think of a time when you felt overwhelmed. What did your body and mind experience?

....

....

....

....

....

6. What usually helps you feel more grounded when stress builds up? How do you feel afterward?

....

....

....

....

....

7. After mentally scanning your body from head to toe, what did you notice—and how did it make you feel?

....

....

....

....

....

Goals and Purpose

1. What do you hope this journal helps you create, shift, or understand over time?

....

....

....

....

....

2. What's one small step you could take this week toward something you've been hoping for?

....

....

....

....

....

3. What did your younger self hope to become—and how close or far have you come?

....

....

....

....

....

4. What tends to slow you down—and what helps reignite your drive?

....

....

....

....

....

5. If there were no limits, what role or job would light you up—and what would your days look like?

....

....

....

....

....

6. If you could visit another time—past or future—what clarity or healing would you seek?

_____

_____

_____

_____

_____

7. What's one thing you can set up now to help next week feel smoother or more purposeful?

_____

_____

_____

_____

_____

Calm and Resiliency

1. What's been on your mind lately? Can writing it down help you set it aside, even just for now?

....

....

....

....

....

2. Choose a word that calms or uplifts you. What might shift if you kept it close today?

....

....

....

....

....

3. Take a slow, steady breath. How do you feel afterward—physically, mentally, emotionally?

....

....

....

....

....

4. What about your body and your being makes you feel grounded, capable, or at peace?

....

....

....

....

....

5. When did you face something hard and come through it? What stayed with you from that moment?

....

....

....

....

....

6. Who could you gently connect with today—and how might that strengthen your sense of support or well-being?

....

....

....

....

....

7. What makes your space feel more peaceful? What small shifts could help you feel more at ease there?

....

....

....

....

....

Connection and Engagement

1. What activities leave you feeling energized and connected? Why does it matter to you?

....

....

....

....

....

2. When did you last feel truly seen or understood by someone? What made that moment special?

....

....

....

....

....

3. Who do you miss connecting with? What gentle steps could bring you closer again?

....

....

....

....

....

4. Have you ever ended up somewhere unexpected—and met someone who made a lasting impact?

....

....

....

....

....

5. What kind words stayed with you—and what did they affirm about who you are?

....

....

....

....

....

6. What shared moments come to mind when you think of joy or closeness? What makes them stand out?

....

....

....

....

....

7. Who would appreciate a kind word from you right now? What would you like to tell them?

....

....

....

....

....

Healthy Living

1. What self-care practices are part of your weekly rhythm? Which ones do you return to most often?

....

....

....

....

....

2. What could make a small area in your home feel more joyful or comforting just for you?

....

....

....

....

....

3. What are five ways you could show up for your health—
emotionally and physically—this month?

....

....

....

....

....

4. What small habit could you introduce today that supports your
happiness or peace of mind?

....

....

....

....

....

5. Looking back at a time when worry took over—what helped
ease it, and what might you do differently now?

....

....

....

....

....

6. What changes or additions would make your home feel more peaceful or supportive?

....

....

....

....

....

7. What's one thing you could do today to clear a little mental space—and why might that help you feel more balanced?

....

....

....

....

....

Goals and Purpose

1. What's one goal you still hold close—and what's been in the way of reaching it so far?

....

....

....

....

....

2. What would it look like to break your goal into small, manageable weekly steps?

....

....

....

....

....

3. Is there a path or passion you've dreamed of exploring? What's one small step you could take toward it?

....

....

....

....

....

4. If this weekend were a chance to reconnect with who you are becoming, what would that look like?

....

....

....

....

....

5. If you had a weekend to recharge anywhere, where would you go and how would you spend it?

....

....

....

....

....

6. What are four joy-filled activities you've missed? How could you reintroduce them over the next month?

....

....

....

....

....

7. What would help you feel more focused and balanced in the week ahead?

....

....

....

....

....

Calm and Resiliency

1. Imagine a morning that feels just right. What elements would make it so—and how can you move closer to that?

....

....

....

....

....

2. What songs lift or ground you? What emotions or memories do they stir?

....

....

....

....

....

3. Reflect on a moment of sadness or worry. What insight came once you made it through?

....

....

....

....

....

4. What's one activity that leaves you feeling truly centered? Describe the experience.

....

....

....

....

....

5. Imagine your favorite color surrounding you. What feelings or memories rise up?

....

....

....

....

....

6. Visualize a peaceful sunrise scene. What do you notice with your senses—and how do you feel in that space?

....

....

....

....

....

7. What helps you keep going when things get tough? Describe the tools or practices that support your resilience.

....

....

....

....

....

Connection and Engagement

1. Imagine a joyful gathering with those who matter to you—who would be there, and how would you spend your time together?

....

....

....

....

....

2. Think of someone who truly uplifts you—what about them brings you lightness or strength?

....

....

....

....

....

3. Who are the most impactful people in your life? What gifts—big or small—have they given you?

....

....

....

....

....

4. What simple act of kindness could you offer soon? How might it shift your day or theirs?

....

....

....

....

....

5. What's an experience you'd love to share with someone—and who would make it even more special?

....

....

....

....

....

6. If you suddenly had the means to give back, who would you support and why?

....

....

....

....

....

7. How could you show up for someone next week? How might that create meaning or connection for you?

....

....

....

....

....

Healthy Living

1. What nourishing foods do you love—and how often do they show up in your week?

....

....

....

....

....

2. How would you rate your daily habits for health and balance? What small changes could improve such a rating?

....

....

....

....

....

3. What's your go-to way to unwind after a long day—and does it truly help you reset?

....

....

....

....

....

4. Take a moment to picture your favorite place. What sensations or emotions rise within you there?

....

....

....

....

....

5. When during the day do you feel most clear, capable, or alive? How do you spend that time?

....

....

....

....

....

6. What drinks refresh or energize you in a healthy way? How could you incorporate them more consistently?

....

....

....

....

....

7. What helps you shift gears when stress builds—what three actions work best for you?

....

....

....

....

....

Goals and Purpose

1. What do you need and hope to accomplish this week? How can you make space for both?

....

....

....

....

....

2. What gives you the strength or reason to carry on each day?

....

....

....

....

....

3. When goals slip through your fingers, what emotions rise—and how do you move through them?

....

....

....

....

....

4. What inner voices or beliefs make it harder to reach your goals?

....

....

....

....

....

5. What strengths or truths can you call on to soften or challenge those limiting thoughts?

....

....

....

....

....

6. What consistently gives you energy, meaning, or drive in your daily life?

....

....

....

....

....

7. What does true success feel or look like for you—and how might that definition be evolving?

....

....

....

....

....

Calm and Resiliency

1. What song brings you a sense of calm or peace? What meaning does it hold for you?

....

....

....

....

....

2. What helps you regain your balance when life knocks you down?

....

....

....

....

....

3. What supportive words would comfort you today if they came from someone who cares? Say them to yourself now.

....

....

....

....

....

4. When did you feel most resilient in the face of a challenge? What helped you get through it?

....

....

....

....

....

5. What kind of weather lifts your mood—and what outdoor moments do you enjoy in it?

....

....

....

....

....

6. What memory from your younger years still brings you warmth or joy?

_____

_____

_____

_____

_____

7. What object nearby holds a positive memory? What story or emotion is attached to it?

_____

_____

_____

_____

_____

Connection and Engagement

1. What shared activities bring you joy or ease when you're with friends?

....

....

....

....

....

2. What moment with someone you love stands out from the past year? What made it special?

....

....

....

....

....

3. What qualities do you admire in someone close—and how do they inspire you?

....

....

....

....

....

4. When you're in need, who do you reach out to—and how have they supported you?

....

....

....

....

....

5. Has someone you trust ever given you advice that stayed with you? How did it help—or not?

....

....

....

....

....

6. How do you imagine your closest friend sees you—inside and out?

....

....

....

....

....

7. Who offered you kindness recently? What feels like a heartfelt way to give it back?

....

....

....

....

....

Healthy Living

1. What simple physical practices—like stretching or breathing—
can you include throughout your day?

....

....

....

....

....

2. After adjusting your posture and breathing deeply, what
changed in your body or mind?

....

....

....

....

....

3. How's your hydration lately? What small changes would help you stay more nourished and refreshed?

....

....

....

....

....

4. How has your sleep been lately—and what might help you feel more rested?

....

....

....

....

....

5. What steps could help you wind down at night in a way that supports deeper rest?

....

....

....

....

....

6. What recent dream left you feeling inspired or energized?
What was it about?

....

....

....

....

....

7. What's your go-to drink—and how does it make you feel,
physically or emotionally?

....

....

....

....

....

Goals and Purpose

1. What's a small but meaningful goal you can set for this week? How might it support your well-being?

....

....

....

....

....

2. What activities bring you a sense of meaning or joy? What do they say about your current purpose?

....

....

....

....

....

3. What would a supportive, organized space look like for you at home? What would make it feel calm and focused?

....

....

....

....

....

4. If money were no object, how might you pursue your purpose differently—and what would stay the same?

....

....

....

....

....

5. If you had one wish to improve your life, what would it be—and how would it impact your well-being?

....

....

....

....

....

6. What three things matter most to complete or honor this week —and what small steps can help you get there?

....

....

....

....

....

7. What parts of your work or hobbies bring you joy—and why do they feel good or fulfilling?

....

....

....

....

....

Calm and Resiliency

1. Think back to a certain age. What's the first memory that surfaces—and how do you feel revisiting it?

....

....

....

....

....

2. Do you feel more at ease by the ocean or in the mountains? What is it about that place that feels calming to you right now?

....

....

....

....

....

3. If you could change something from the past, what would it be —and how might life feel different today?

....

....

....

....

....

4. What kind of weather brings you peace—and what does that calm feel like in your body or mind?

....

....

....

....

....

5. What songs lift your mood or remind you of your strength? List the ones that bring you back to yourself.

....

....

....

....

....

6. What's one thing that's going well for you right now—and what emotions does that bring up?

....

....

....

....

....

7. What's something simple and enjoyable you could plan for next week—and how might you make space to enjoy it more than once?

....

....

....

....

....

Connection and Engagement

1. Who brings lightness and joy into your life? What do they do that lifts your spirit?

....

....

....

....

....

2. Imagine planning a celebration for your closest friend. What theme would reflect their essence?

....

....

....

....

....

3. If you had a travel companion for your dream trip, who would it be—and what makes them your first choice?

....

....

....

....

....

4. What kinds of talks leave you feeling seen and connected?

....

....

....

....

....

5. What nearby places feel meaningful or energizing to you when shared with others?

....

....

....

....

....

6. What artist or band would you love to see live—and what part of the experience would lift you up?

....

....

....

....

....

7. What five words describe someone you admire? What do those words say about who they are to you?

....

....

....

....

....

Healthy Living

1. What did the sky look like today—and how did it affect your mood or thoughts?

....

....

....

....

....

2. How do you currently view yourself—and is there a shift you're hoping for?

....

....

....

....

....

3. If your life were structured like an athlete's, what sport would suit you—and what healthy habits would be essential?

....

....

....

....

....

4. What sensations or emotions did you notice during your most recent movement outdoors?

....

....

....

....

....

5. How do food and movement fit into your idea of self-care or wellness?

....

....

....

....

....

6. What feelings come up when you think about your relationship with food? What would you like to shift?

....

....

....

....

....

7. What would a day of full, balanced health feel like for you—physically and emotionally?

....

....

....

....

....

Goals and Purpose

1. Have you done something kind for someone close to you lately? How did it affect them—or you?

....

....

....

....

....

2. What 10 actions, big or small, could brighten someone's day or life?

....

....

....

....

....

3. What lasting impact or memory would you like to leave behind?

....

....

....

....

....

4. If forced to choose, which feels more valuable to you—abundance or well-being?

....

....

....

....

....

5. What three things would give you a sense of progress or purpose this week?

....

....

....

....

....

6. What past success means the most to you—and what makes it so meaningful?

....

....

....

....

....

7. What kind of museum would you enjoy visiting—and who would you want beside you to share that experience?

....

....

....

....

....

Calm and Resiliency

1. What five things help you feel calm when you're upset—and how might you use them more intentionally?

....

....

....

....

....

2. Without a phone for a day, what would you spend your time doing instead—and how might it feel?

....

....

....

....

....

3. After three quiet minutes, what thoughts rose to the surface? What might they reveal?

....

....

....

....

....

4. What uplifts your mood when you're low? What does it feel like afterward?

....

....

....

....

....

5. Picture yourself near water. What sensory details stand out— and what feelings arise?

....

....

....

....

....

6. Fill in the blank: Today I feel good about myself because...

....

....

....

....

....

7. When have you felt fear—but moved forward anyway? What helped you do it?

....

....

....

....

....

Connection and Engagement

1. What shared activities with coworkers or peers bring you enjoyment or ease?

....

....

....

....

....

2. How might you contribute or connect more with your community in a way that feels good to you?

....

....

....

....

....

3. Picture walking by the water with a close friend—what kinds of conversations might unfold?

_____

_____

_____

_____

_____

4. Who was your first real friend—and what made that connection special or memorable?

_____

_____

_____

_____

_____

5. What stood out about your last visit to the movies or a live performance—aside from what you watched?

_____

_____

_____

_____

_____

6. What joyful moment from early school years do you still remember fondly?

....

....

....

....

....

7. Imagine a journey to a magical place. Who joins you—and how do you spend your time there?

....

....

....

....

....

Healthy Living

1. If you could learn a new language, which one calls to you and where might you use it?

....

....

....

....

....

2. Is there a show that lifts your mood or helps you relax? What about it feels comforting to you?

....

....

....

....

....

3. Where would your ideal cruise take you—and what joyful activities would fill your time?

....

....

....

....

....

4. When did you last feel truly balanced and well? What habits supported you then?

....

....

....

....

....

5. What clothes help you feel most like yourself? What do they express about you?

....

....

....

....

....

6. What do you love capturing in photos—and how might that shift with a professional camera?

....

....

....

....

....

7. After a long week, what helps you unwind or reset?

....

....

....

....

....

Goals and Purpose

1. Imagine your future self five years from now. What goals will you be proud to have reached?

....

....

....

....

....

2. How do you feel emotionally and physically when you reflect on your biggest win?

....

....

....

....

....

3. What's one thing you feel thankful for today—and how does it shape your outlook?

....

....

....

....

....

4. Imagine visiting a peaceful planet. What would you explore— and how might it reflect your inner world?

....

....

....

....

....

5. Without financial limits, what purpose would guide your days— and who would it touch?

....

....

....

....

....

6. Who taught you something you still carry? What would you want to thank them for now?

_____

_____

_____

_____

_____

7. If your dream job took you somewhere new, what would the work and home look like?

_____

_____

_____

_____

_____

Calm and Resiliency

1. What five ways help you cope when life gets tough?

....

....

....

....

....

2. What happens in your body and mind when you confront fear?

....

....

....

....

....

3. What calming thoughts or actions remind you that you can keep going during hard moments?

....

....

....

....

....

4. What types of situations test your patience—and what thoughts tend to show up in those moments?

....

....

....

....

....

5. Reflect on a tough day. What emotions took hold—and what helped bring relief or light?

....

....

....

....

....

6. What five activities bring you calm—and how lasting is that peace afterward?

....

....

....

....

....

7. When plans fall through, what emotions and thoughts come up for you?

....

....

....

....

....

Connection and Engagement

1. What act of kindness from someone else has stayed with you—and why?

....

....

....

....

....

2. What made you laugh recently—and what did that laughter feel like in your body?

....

....

....

....

....

3. What would a meaningful, easeful day with someone close look like?

....

....

....

....

....

4. What would you say in a thank-you note to someone who showed you care recently?

....

....

....

....

....

5. What five questions could open up real conversation when meeting someone new?

....

....

....

....

....

6. Who's an old friend you'd love to reconnect with—and what would that day look like?

....

....

....

....

....

7. What would a connection-filled, joyful date feel like—with someone you love or hope to meet?

....

....

....

....

....

Healthy Living

1. How are you feeling today in mind, heart, and body? What might help you feel a little better?

....

....

....

....

....

2. Which kind of weather feels more comforting or energizing to you—sunny or overcast—and why?

....

....

....

....

....

3. What meals or snacks give your body and spirit a lift?

....

....

....

....

4. What would your ideal rest space look and feel like?

....

....

....

....

5. If one fitness space could be yours, which would best support your well-being—and why?

....

....

....

....

6. What three things would you explore if fear didn't hold you back?

....

....

....

....

....

7. What does a "good week" feel like in your body, thoughts, and emotions?

....

....

....

....

....

Goals and Purpose

1. What helps you stay focused on a goal—and why does it matter to you?

....

....

....

....

....

2. What helps you return to steadiness when fear or anxiety shows up?

....

....

....

....

....

3. If you had the power to heal one emotional struggle, which would you choose—and why?

....

....

....

....

....

4. What three past goals have you met—and what supported you on the journey?

....

....

....

....

....

5. What dream or aim would mean the most for you to fulfill in your life?

....

....

....

....

....

6. What thoughts, circumstances, or habits feel like barriers to your goals—and how might they shift?

....

....

....

....

....

7. What words of care and encouragement would you offer a friend on the edge of a leap?

....

....

....

....

....

Calm and Resiliency

1. What's a favorite show you've returned to over the years—and why does it stay with you?

....

....

....

....

....

2. What type of moment stirs anxiety for you—and what practice helps ease it?

....

....

....

....

....

3. What top stressors showed up this week—and how might you handle them differently next time?

....

....

....

....

....

4. Write a short message to your stress—letting it know you're reclaiming peace.

....

....

....

....

....

5. Think of a recent challenge. What helped you feel steady again afterward?

....

....

....

....

....

6. What would your ideal workspace look like if it helped you feel calm, clear, and focused?

....

....

....

....

....

7. Which songs make you feel stronger or bolder? What do they awaken in you?

....

....

....

....

....

Connection and Engagement

1. What are five things you think your close friend enjoys—and how aligned is your guess?

....

....

....

....

....

2. If you had a gift card just for giving—what would you choose and who would it be for?

....

....

....

....

....

3. Imagine a 24-hour airport chat with someone well-known. Who is it—and what do you talk about?

....

....

....

....

....

4. What does your circle of support do that helps you feel safe or valued?

....

....

....

....

....

5. What weekend plans would feel meaningful or fun with someone close to you?

....

....

....

....

....

6. What would you say in a heartfelt apology to someone you've wronged?

_____

_____

_____

_____

_____

7. What would an ideal day of connection in your community look like?

_____

_____

_____

_____

_____

Healthy Living

1. What usually helps lift your mood when you're feeling low?

....

....

....

....

....

2. What does your ideal lunch look like, and how does it make you feel?

....

....

....

....

....

3. How do you care for your body with food each day? What feels worth adjusting?

_____

_____

_____

_____

_____

4. How is your sleep lately? What would help you feel more rested?

_____

_____

_____

_____

_____

5. What kinds of movement make you feel energized and alive?

_____

_____

_____

_____

_____

6. Imagine a superhero with your best qualities—what are they like?

....

....

....

....

....

7. What's one step today that moves you closer to your most empowered self?

....

....

....

....

....

Goals and Purpose

1. What feels like it's working or flowing well for you right now?

....

....

....

....

....

2. What feels hard right now? How can you reframe it with possibility or compassion?

....

....

....

....

....

3. What image brings you joy when you see it? What feelings come up?

....

....

....

....

....

4. What small strategies help you stay grounded and intentional with your goals?

....

....

....

....

....

5. Imagine your ideal day. What's one way you can bring part of it into tomorrow?

....

....

....

....

....

6. What growth goals are important to you—and what steps could support them?

....

....

....

....

....

7. How do you make everyday moments feel meaningful or memorable?

....

....

....

....

....

Calm and Resiliency

1. What local spots help you feel at ease or grounded?

....

....

....

....

....

2. Where in your home do you feel most at peace? How could you enhance that space?

....

....

....

....

....

3. What object in your home holds deep meaning for you—and what's the story behind it?

....

....

....

....

....

4. After a few deep breaths, what thought or memory helps you feel at peace?

....

....

....

....

....

5. When you're joyful, how do others see or experience you?

....

....

....

....

....

6. What colors do you wear that help you feel calm or confident?

....

....

....

....

....

7. After your last cry, what shifted inside you? What did the release feel like?

....

....

....

....

....

Connection and Engagement

1. Who are two people you feel closest to—and what is it about them that makes their presence so meaningful?

....

....

....

....

....

2. Who do you turn to when you're feeling low? What helps in the way they show up for you?

....

....

....

....

....

3. What shared activities lift your spirits or ease anxiety when you're not feeling your best?

....

....

....

....

....

4. What shared moments or experiences would bring you and a friend more joy this month?

....

....

....

....

....

5. What's a personal milestone you'd like to reach with someone's support—and how can you start?

....

....

....

....

....

6. Who are five people who matter to you—and how can you show them they're valued?

....

....

....

....

....

7. Who have you lost touch with that you'd like to reconnect with? What would you say to them now?

....

....

....

....

....

Healthy Living

1. How would you rate your sleep lately? What's helping or getting in the way?

....

....

....

....

....

2. What task drains your energy right now—and how might you lighten the load or reframe it?

....

....

....

....

....

3. How does different weather affect your mood or energy?

....

....

....

....

....

4. What new interest calls to you—and how might it bring energy or joy?

....

....

....

....

....

5. What's been on your mind lately? How might you begin to ease or address it?

....

....

....

....

....

6. Which day feels best for you—and what about it helps you feel good?

....

....

....

....

....

7. What's something you enjoy doing on a day like this—and what makes it satisfying?

....

....

....

....

....

Goals and Purpose

1. What feels like a meaningful goal to focus on this week?

....

....

....

....

....

2. Is there a phrase or belief that helps you feel grounded or encouraged? How could you keep it closer in your daily life?

....

....

....

....

....

3. What's one area of life you wish felt more manageable? What difference would that make?

....

....

....

....

....

4. Who would you meet for a meaningful lunch—and what ideas or questions would you bring?

....

....

....

....

....

5. What shift would you love to see in your neighborhood or city— and can you contribute to it?

....

....

....

....

....

6. How might you invest more care or intention in the relationships that matter to you?

....

....

....

....

....

7. What upcoming plans help you feel excited or purposeful—and why?

....

....

....

....

....

Healthy Living

1. When your mind races ahead, what helps bring you back to now?

....

....

....

....

....

2. What helps ease your stress when life feels heavy?

....

....

....

....

....

3. What helped you through a moment of intense fear or panic in the past?

....

....

....

....

....

4. What life experience pushed you to grow stronger? What did you learn from it?

....

....

....

....

....

5. What piece of clothing helps you feel most like yourself?

....

....

....

....

....

6. What simple act could you do today to help someone feel more at peace?

....

....

....

....

....

7. What was one uplifting moment from your week that you'd love to experience again?

....

....

....

....

....

Connection and Engagement

1. Who do you miss spending time with lately? What would reconnecting look like?

....

....

....

....

....

2. Who helps you feel safe just by being around—and what do they do that grounds you?

....

....

....

....

....

3. What was the last conversation you had with someone close to you—and what part of it stayed with you?

....

....

....

....

....

4. Do you tend to connect more with upbeat or more reserved friends? What draws you in?

....

....

....

....

....

5. What's something you enjoy doing with someone else that helps lift your mood on tough days?

....

....

....

....

....

6. What gift has touched you most deeply—and what gift have you loved giving?

....

....

....

....

....

7. What's a memory with a friend that still makes you laugh?

....

....

....

....

....

Healthy Living

1. What are five actions that support your mental well-being?

....

....

....

....

....

2. Recall a recent high-stress moment. What contributed to the pressure?

....

....

....

....

....

3. What recent activity boosted your health and happiness?

....

....

....

....

....

4. Which past healthy habits have you maintained or let go?

....

....

....

....

....

5. Who motivates you to grow? How would a day with them unfold?

....

....

....

....

....

6. What strategies help you choose health during emotional lows?

....

....

....

....

....

7. Are there thoughts holding you back from your wellness goals?

....

....

....

....

....

Goals and Purpose

1. What's one change today that could ease your week?

....

....

....

....

....

2. What affirmations could support you during unexpected challenges?

....

....

....

....

....

3. Among your goals, which feels most pressing right now?

_____

_____

_____

_____

4. Envision yourself in two years. What are you doing?

_____

_____

_____

_____

5. What guidance would you offer someone pursuing a goal?

_____

_____

_____

_____

6. What simple additions could enrich your daily routines?

....

....

....

....

....

7. What's a purposeful goal you can set for the coming week?

....

....

....

....

....

Calm and Resiliency

1. What techniques help you regain calm during overwhelm?

....

....

....

....

....

2. What can you decline this week to honor your well-being?

....

....

....

....

....

3. What steps can you take to make your home more peaceful?

....

....

....

....

....

4. Which scenarios trigger your anxiety? How do you cope?

....

....

....

....

....

5. What free activity would bring you joy tomorrow afternoon?

....

....

....

....

....

Calm and Resiliency

6. Reflect on your resilience. What makes you proud?

....

....

....

....

....

7. Which recent actions boosted your self-esteem?

....

....

....

....

....

Connection and Engagement

1. What steps can enhance your self-relationship?

....

....

....

....

....

2. Which interpersonal skills can you focus on to build connections?

....

....

....

....

....

3. How can you meaningfully honor your loved ones?

....

....

....

....

....

4. In what ways can you lend support to others?

....

....

....

....

....

5. Which shared experiences with friends bring you joy?

....

....

....

....

....

6. How can you enhance the balance in your friendships?

....

....

....

....

....

7. What wellness practices can you share with loved ones?

....

....

....

....

....

Healthy Living

1. What boundaries help you manage stress and protect your peace?

....

....

....

....

....

2. How do you maintain your well-being around people who feel emotionally heavy?

....

....

....

....

....

3. Reflect on a time in your life when you felt your best. What habits made that possible?

....

....

....

....

....

4. What would a nourishing meal plan look like for you this week?

....

....

....

....

....

5. What daily practices help you feel whole—body, mind, and spirit?

....

....

....

....

....

6. What keeps you resilient in the face of negativity or outside pressure?

....

....

....

....

....

7. If you've been trying to care for yourself in healthier ways, what comforting alternatives have been helping?

....

....

....

....

....

Goals and Purpose

1. What does living with purpose mean to you today?

....

....

....

....

....

2. What two life experiences have shaped your sense of meaning or direction?

....

....

....

....

....

3. What's one small step you could take this weekend toward a meaningful goal?

....

....

....

....

....

4. What achievement—no matter how small—has made you smile lately?

....

....

....

....

....

5. What did you follow through on this week that left you feeling accomplished?

....

....

....

....

....

6. Of all your current goals, which one matters most to you right now—and why?

....

....

....

....

....

7. What's a practical, manageable way to move toward your goal this week?

....

....

....

....

....

Calm and Resiliency

1. Describe a calming place that made you feel deeply at peace.

....

....

....

....

....

2. What helps your body and mind settle before sleep?

....

....

....

....

....

3. Recall a dream that left you feeling joyful or peaceful.

....

....

....

....

....

4. Think of a recent happy moment. What brought that feeling into your day?

....

....

....

....

....

5. How did you find your footing during a tough moment?

....

....

....

....

....

6. Which songs help you feel calm and clear?

....

....

....

....

....

7. What helps you recover when things go wrong? What shaped that strength?

....

....

....

....

....

Connection and Engagement

1. What's one meaningful way you can strengthen a close relationship in your life?

....

....

....

....

....

2. Is there someone you'd like to forgive, even just a little? What might that first step look like?

....

....

....

....

....

3. If you're feeling resentful, what boundaries or reflections might help you move toward peace?

_____

_____

_____

_____

_____

4. Who inspires you to be your best self? What qualities do they reflect?

_____

_____

_____

_____

_____

5. Who are three people you deeply appreciate, and what makes their impact so meaningful?

_____

_____

_____

_____

_____

6. How might you express your gratitude to those people in a way that feels genuine?

....

....

....

....

....

7. What issue or cause stirs your heart? How could you get involved or show your support?

....

....

....

....

....

Healthy Living

1. What's weighing on your to-do list, and how can you take care of yourself while handling it?

....

....

....

....

....

2. How does your mental well-being show up in your everyday life —and how do you care for it?

....

....

....

....

....

3. How is your mind and mood today? What do you need more—
or less—of?

....

....

....

....

....

4. What's something on your mind that you'd feel relieved to talk
to a therapist about?

....

....

....

....

....

5. How would you describe your views on therapy if someone you
care about asked for your thoughts?

....

....

....

....

....

6. What emotions are present for you right now? Are any taking up more space than others?

....

....

....

....

....

7. Why does your emotional well-being matter to you? What would you want to tell yourself about that?

....

....

....

....

....

Goals and Purpose

1. What's changed for you over the past few years—and what do you think influenced those shifts?

....

....

....

....

....

2. What quote gives you strength or hope—and why does it speak to you?

....

....

....

....

....

3. When something gets in the way of a goal, how do you process or respond?

....

....

....

....

....

4. What did the past year teach you about your values or what truly matters?

....

....

....

....

....

5. Is there a story you've been meaning to explore—on a page or a screen? What's pulling you toward it?

....

....

....

....

....

6. What could you complete this weekend that would feel both doable and meaningful?

....

....

....

....

....

7. What kind of service would feel meaningful to offer your community—if you had the time?

....

....

....

....

....

Calm and Resiliency

1. What's one limiting thought that's ready to be released? What might help you release it?

....

....

....

....

....

2. Think back to a time you felt anxious. What did it feel like in your body and mind—and what might you try now?

....

....

....

....

....

3. If someone who cares about you heard your inner worries, what words might they offer?

....

....

....

....

....

4. When you take a deep breath, how does it shift your body and thoughts? Do you practice this often?

....

....

....

....

....

5. What fears still sit with you? What have you done—or could do —to ease their hold?

....

....

....

....

....

6. Are your fears grounded in fact or imagination? What do you know to be true?

....

....

....

....

....

7. What helps calm your mind when it feels overactive? What practices have you found helpful or want to try?

....

....

....

....

....

Connection and Engagement

1. What are five ways you could nurture the important relationships in your life?

....

....

....

....

....

2. What boundaries would protect your well-being in draining relationships?

....

....

....

....

....

3. When is it hard to say "no"? What might make it easier for you to hold your limits with care?

....

....

....

....

....

4. What small actions or gestures bring joy to those around you?

....

....

....

....

....

5. When anticipating a tough talk, what can help calm your nerves and keep you grounded?

....

....

....

....

....

6. Who's a fictional character you admire? What about them inspires action or courage in you?

....

....

....

....

....

7. What are five enjoyable ways to spend time with your family in the near future?

....

....

....

....

....

Healthy Living

1. What challenges made healthy living harder this past year?

....

....

....

....

....

2. How did you respond to those challenges, and what helped you move forward?

....

....

....

....

....

3. How are your mind and emotions doing today? Be honest and gentle in your reflection.

....

....

....

....

....

4. What's one way you'll stay committed to your well-being in the year ahead?

....

....

....

....

....

5. What role has journaling played in your emotional or mental clarity this year?

....

....

....

....

....

6. What forms of movement do you want to try or return to—and what draws you to them?

....

....

....

....

....

7. What habits or mindsets might help you stay steady when life gets stressful?

....

....

....

....

....

Goals and Purpose

1. Reflect on your latest wins. What makes you proud—and what strength did it take to get there?

....

....

....

....

....

2. What's a dream you'd love to bring to life next year?

....

....

....

....

....

3. What's the first step you can take toward a goal that matters to you right now?

....

....

....

....

....

4. How have you grown or changed since you began this journaling journey?

....

....

....

....

....

5. What are five affirming phrases that will support your well-being beyond this journal?

....

....

....

....

....

6. What are the top five things you've discovered, accomplished, or reclaimed since starting this journal?

....

....

....

....

....

7. You've completed a year of showing up for yourself. What do you want to say in celebration?

....

....

....

....

....

Keep Growing, Keep Asking:
Discover More Titles

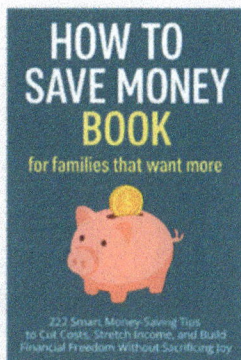

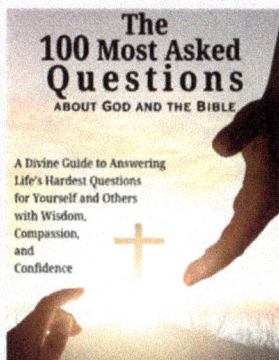

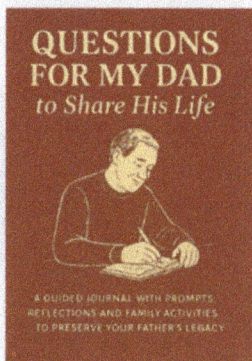

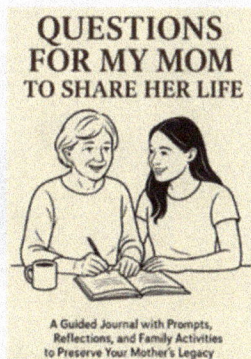

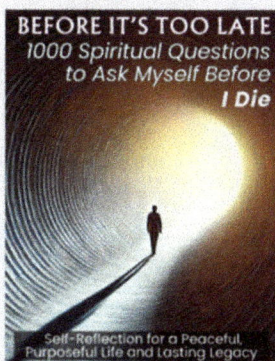

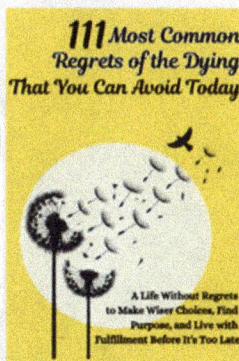

HOW TO SAVE MONEY BOOK
for families that want more

222 Smart Money-Saving Tips to Cut Costs, Stretch Income, and Build Financial Freedom Without Sacrificing Joy

The 100 Most Asked Questions
ABOUT GOD AND THE BIBLE

A Divine Guide to Answering Life's Hardest Questions for Yourself and Others with Wisdom, Compassion, and Confidence

QUESTIONS FOR MY DAD
to Share His Life

A GUIDED JOURNAL WITH PROMPTS, REFLECTIONS AND FAMILY ACTIVITIES TO PRESERVE YOUR FATHER'S LEGACY

QUESTIONS FOR MY MOM
TO SHARE HER LIFE

A Guided Journal with Prompts, Reflections, and Family Activities to Preserve Your Mother's Legacy

BEFORE IT'S TOO LATE
1000 Spiritual Questions to Ask Myself Before I Die

Self-Reflection for a Peaceful, Purposeful Life and Lasting Legacy

111 Most Common Regrets of the Dying That You Can Avoid Today

A Life Without Regrets to Make Wiser Choices, Find Purpose, and Live with Fulfillment Before It's Too Late

www.ingramcontent.com/pod-product-compliance
Lightning Source LLC
Chambersburg PA
CBHW070113030426
42335CB00016B/2141